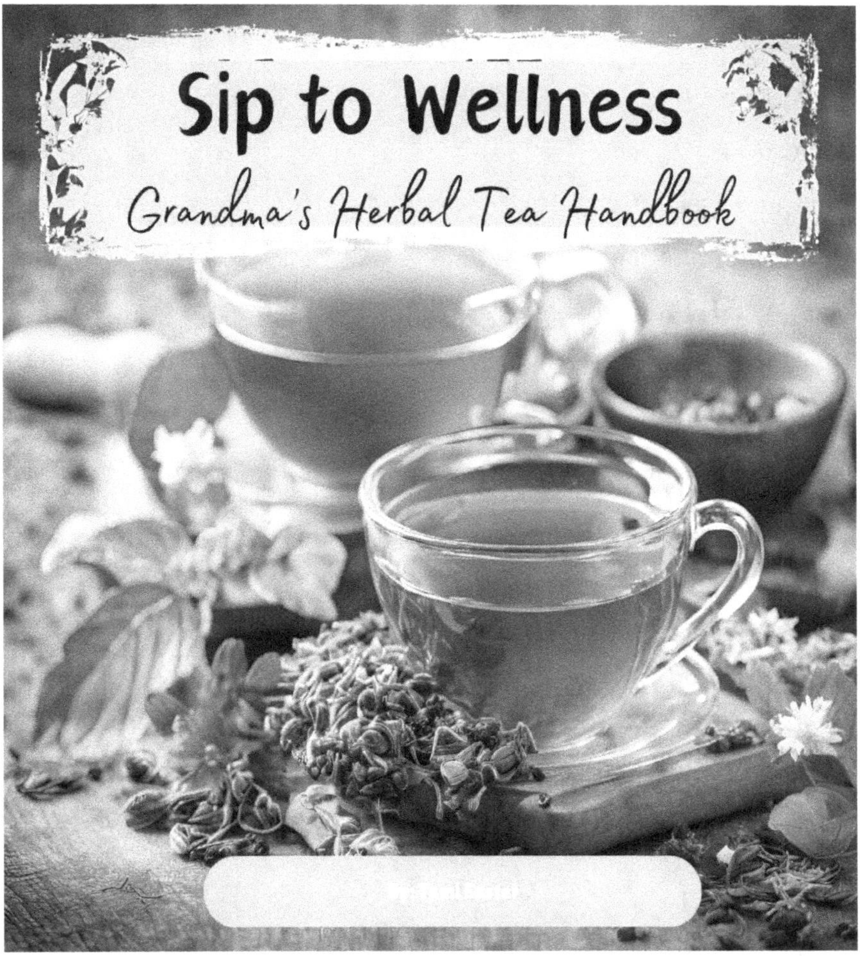

Sip to Wellness

Grandma's Herbal Tea Handbook

Table of Contents

Disclaimer

I am simply a human looking for answers in my continual search for natural remedies to my own medical ailments. These ailments have caused me chronic pain, fatigue, gastric/stomach problems, skin issues, and so-on. I have found some things helpful. Some, not so much.

What I am not is a physician, or medical professional. Information provided is not designed to diagnose, prescribe, or treat any illness, or injury and is provided for informational purposes only.

Be aware that each individual is different and their body may react differently to certain herbs. Just as with a food allergy a person may have a personal reaction to an herb that is not necessarily a toxic substance. Although these are natural products they may become toxic if misused.

These herbal uses and properties are only given for reference purposes. If you're unsure of what the correct uses and doSages of herbs to be used are please consult an Ayurevic, or holistic practitioner.

I am not responsible for any actions or outcome of use of these remedies taken by persons using these references. I ask that you please consult your physician before adding or changing any dietary or herbal supplements to your diet.

Dedication

In loving dedication to Edith M Bowen (Mommy) to me, and (Grandma) to many. Not only did you pass down a genetic lottery! You have also given the wisdom of understanding the power held in the foods we eat.

May you continue to live on forever!

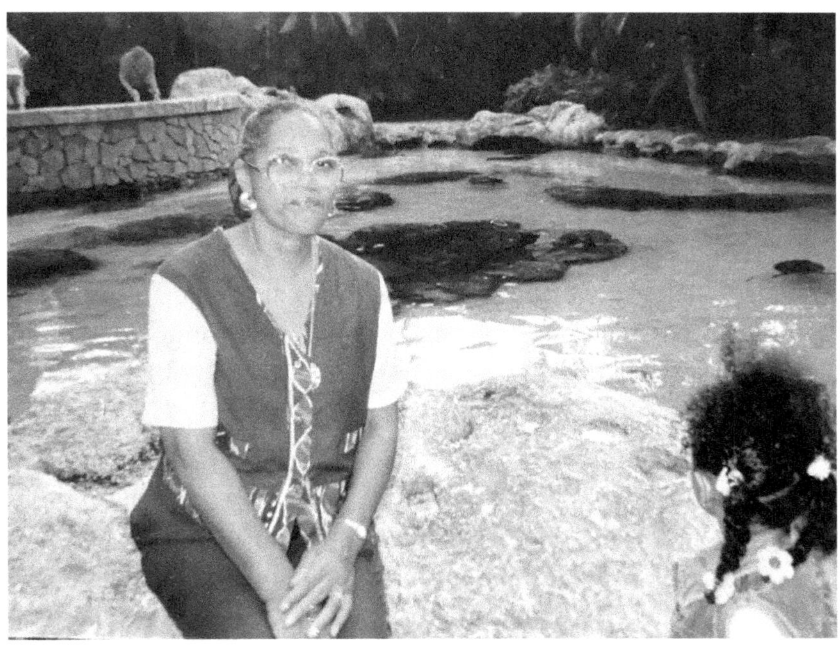

Tea Time

True tea only comes from one plant: *Camellia sinensis*. Black, green, white, and oolong may look and taste different, but the only real difference is how long the leaves oxidize before they're dried. That oxidation changes everything—from flavor to color to antioxidant strength.

These teas come loose or in tea bags, depending on how fancy you're feeling.

Herbal teas (a.k.a. tisanes) aren't technically tea. They're brewed from herbs, spices, flowers, and roots like chamomile, hibiscus, peppermint, ginger, or turmeric. Most people use dried ingredients, but fresh herbs work beautifully too.

While the method is similar, steeping times and water temps aren't one-size-fits-all. Steeping pulls out flavor, scent, antioxidants, and caffeine. Hot tea needs only a few minutes to brew; cold tea takes 8–12 hours but tastes smoother and often contains more antioxidants.

Research shows black tea hits peak antioxidant power around the 6–8 minute mark. And yes—more time equals more caffeine. A 6 oz cup of black tea averages about 35 mg of caffeine, compared to 21 mg in green tea. Every extra minute of steeping can bump caffeine by nearly 30%, and boiling water can boost it even more.

❊ ✳ ☕ ✳ ❊

21st Century Tea

There are so many ways that our immune systems can be overwhelmed ... it's in our air, our water, our food, our workplace, our stress. This blend of organic and wild herbs is not only helpful but comforting, strengthening and tasty.

1 pt Red Clover Blossoms
1 pt Nettle Leaves
1 pt Pau d'Arco
1 pt Alfalfa
1 pt Sage leaves
1 pt St. John's Wort tops
1 pt Ginger root

Place all herbs in a tea ball or bag, and cover with boiling water. Steep for 10 minutes.Remove tea ball or bag, and add sugar, honey, sweetener, milk,cream or whatever, to taste.

Aches and Pains Tea

1 tbls. White Willow Bark
1 tbls. Catnip

Put in a tea ball and steep in boiling hot water for five minutes.Drink as hot as you can stand it, then lie down for a nap.

ADD/ADHD Remedy

1 tsp Hops
1 tsp Gotu Kola

Bring 1 1/2 cups of water to a boil. Place the herbs inside, place lid on tightly and let it steep for 5 minutes. Drink twice a day.

After Dinner Carminative Tea

1 cup water
1 tbls. Fennel Seeds

Bring covered pot of water and fennel seeds to a boil and let sit for 15 minutes and enjoy this calming cup of tea. Fennel is a wonderful herb for digestion and can help your body increase its ability to digest a big meal or a meal with lots of fat.

❧ ✳ ☕ ✳ ❧

Allergy Season Blend

Cool minty, citrus flavor to assist you with the discomfort associated with allergy season.

1 pt Nettle
1 pt Peppermint
1 pt Spearmint
1 pt Yerba Santa
1 pt Eyebright
1 pt Lemongrass leaves
1 pt Calendula
1 pt Red Clover
1 pt Lavender flowers 1 pt Fennel Seeds a pinch of stevia

Place all herbs in a tea ball or bag, and cover with boiling water. Steep for 10 minutes.

Remove tea ball or bag, and add sugar, honey, sweetener, milk, cream or whatever, to taste.

Aphrodite Blend Tea

A sensuous, aromatic blend with just the right tint of zest for your palate, and sure to kindle flames! A delicate, but dashing combination makes this one of your most enjoyable cups of tea.

1 pt Damiana leaves
1 pt Rose petals
1 pt Peppermint leaves
1 pt Muira Puama
1 pt Ginkgo leaves
1 pt Orange Peel
1 pt Cinnamon Bark Chips pinch of stevia.

Place all herbs in a tea ball or bag, and cover with boiling water. Steep for 10 minutes.

Remove tea ball or bag, and add sugar, honey, sweetener, milk,cream or whatever, to taste.

Baby Sleep Tea

1 tsp Hops
1 tsp Chamomile

Bring 4 cups of water to a boil. Remove pot from heat and add the herbs. Put a tight lid on the pot and let it steep for five minutes. Strain herbs. Place in four ounce glass bottle once cooled enough for the baby to drink.

***This remedy is not for babies under 6 months old**

Bladder Infections Tea

1 ½ oz dried Goldenrod
1/4 oz Juniper Berries*
3/4 oz chopped Dandelion root
3/4 oz chopped Muira Puama Hips

Pour 1 cup boiling water over 2 tsp of mixture. Steep 10 minutes & strain.
can become toxic, so only drink 2 cups of this mixture daily for no more than 3 days

Blood Builder Tea

1 tsp Rose Hips-crushed
1 Tsp Butcher's Broom
1 Tsp Yellow Dock

Bring 31/2 cups of water to a boil. Remove water from heat and add herbs. Place a tight lid on the pot. Let the mixture steep for five to ten minutes. Drink one cup three times daily. Yields three cups.

Blossoms of Health Tea

Beautiful to look at, nectar to taste and good for you. A popular tea. Spirited, uplifting and energizing.

1 pt Ginkgo leaves
1 pt Red Clover tops
1 pt Nettle Leaves
1 pt meadowsweet leaves
1 pt Calendula
2 pts Chamomile
2 pts Lavender flowers 1 pt Gotu Kola leaves a pinch of stevia.

Place all herbs in a tea ball or bag and cover with boiling water. Steep for 10 minutes. Remove tea ball or bag, and add sugar, honey, sweetener, milk, cream or whatever, to taste.

Blues Tea

1 pt Nettle Leaves,
1 pt St John's wort tops
2 pts Spearmint
1 pt damiana leaves 1 pt Kava Kava root a tiny pinch of stevia to taste

Place all herbs in a tea ball or bag,and cover with boiling water. Steep for 10 minutes. Remove tea ball or bag, and add sugar, honey, sweetener, milk, cream or whatever, to taste.

❊ ✳ ☕ ✳ ❊

Breast Health Tea

2 pts Calendula
2 pts Red Clover
1 pt Cleavers
1 pt Lady's Mantle
Spearmint or Peppermint (optional; for flavor)

Prepare as an infusion, using 1 ounce of herbs per quart of water, and letting it steep overnight. Drink 3 to 4 cups daily.

Bronchial Congestion Tea

1 ½ oz Aniseed
1 oz Calendula flowers
3/4 oz Marshmallow root
1/3 oz Licorice root

Crush anise seeds and add to herbs. Pour 1 cup boiling water over 1 tsp mixture; cover & steep 10 minutes.

Calming Tea 1

1 oz Lemon balm
1 oz Chamomile flowers
½ oz St John's Wort

Steep 2 tbs of mixture in 1 cup boiled water. Cover 10 minutes; strain.

Calming Tea 2

1 pt Sage
1 pt Thyme
1 pt Marjoram
1 pt Chamomile

Blend ingredients in a tea ball and put in a mug of hot water

Colds and Flu Tea

1 oz Blackberry leaves
1 oz Elderflowers
1 oz Linden flowers
1 oz Peppermint leaves

Pour 1 cup boiling water over 2 tbs mixture. Cover & steep 10 minutes; strain.

Colds and Hoarseness Tea

2 oz Malva flowers
1 ½ oz Mullein flowers

Use 2 tbs of mixture per 1 cup hot water. Steep 10 minutes; strain.
Drink only 2 - 3 cups per day for just a few days.

Cold or sinus season Tea

1/4 cup dried Thyme
1/4 cup dried Feverfew flowers
3/4 cup dried Peppermint leaves
1 tbls. dried and rubbed or crushed Sage

Place all herbs in a tea ball or bag, add lemon wedge and cover with boiling water. Steep for 5- 10 minutes.

❀ ✳ ☕ ✳ ❀

Cold Stopper Tea

1 1/2 tbls.s of Licorice root already brewed in a pot enough for two cups.
1 Elderberry tea bag
1 tbls. Chamomile

Steep the tea bag in the Licorice Root infusion and add in the chamomile. This can be done in the coffee maker, but the Licorice brew must be cool enough to be cycled through the machine.

Constipation Tea

1/2 tsp Cáscara Sagrada
1 tsp Chamomile

Place all herbs in a tea ball or bag, add lemon wedge and cover with boiling water. Steep for 10 minutes. Take in one dose before bedtime. One full cup should do it.

Coughing Fits Tea

1 1/3 oz. St. John's Wort
2/3 oz. Thyme
2/3 oz. Linden Flowers

Use 1 tsp. of the herb mixture per cup of boiling water to soothe irritations of the upper respiratory tract that cause coughing. Steep for 5-10 min., strain, sweeten if necessary. This tea has proved helpful with bronchitis and whooping cough.

Cramp Tea

1 tsp Cramp Bark
1 tsp Red Raspberry Leaves
1 tsp Dong Quai

Place all herbs in a tea ball or bag, add lemon wedge and cover with boiling water.Steep for 5- 10 minutes.Take this tea by the cup-fulls. This makes enough for two cups. The tea is only good for six hours.

Crone Root Tea

For menopause and beginning a new cycle of life.

2 tbls.s Wild Yam
2 tbls.s Licorice
3 tbls.s Sarsaparilla
1 tbls. Chaste Berry
1 tbls. Ginger
1 tbls. False Unicorn Root
2 tbls.s Sage
1 tbls. Cinnamon
½ tbls. Black Cohosh

Place all herbs in a tea ball or bag, and cover with boiling water. Steep for 5-10 minutes.

Depression Tamer Tea

1 tsp St John's Wort
1 tsp Ginkgo Biloba

Place 1 cup of water into a glass or porcelain pot and bring to a boil. Remove pot from heat and add the herbs. Put a tight lid on the pot and let it steep for five minutes. Strain out herbals. Place in a cup and sweeten with honey if desired.

Dry, raspy cough

1 tbls. Licorice Root
1 tbls. Slippery Elm
1 tbls. Mullein
1 tbls. Catnip
1 tbls. Chamomile
1 tbls. Honey
1 Lemon wedge

Place all herbs in a tea ball or bag, add lemon wedge and cover with boiling water. Steep for 5-10 minutes.

Detox Tea

1 tsp Pau d'Arco (Taheebo)
1 tsp Cáscara Sagrada
1 tsp Echinacea

Bring 1 1/2 cups water to a boil. Place herbs into the water, cover tightly and let steep for five minutes. I cup two times a day should help. If bowels are loose, dilute the combination in 2 to 2 1/2 cups water.

Dry Congestion Tea

(For thick congestion and irritated mucous membranes.)

2 pts Eyebright
1 pt Catnip
2 pts Thyme
1 pt Goldenrod

Steep 1-1/2 to 2 tsp in a larger cup, such as a coffee mug, for 10 minutes. You will likely need lemon or honey, as this remedy is rather bitter. Very soothing. Try to stay warm while drinking, and for a time afterwards.

**If you experience any discomfort or unpleasant effects while drinking this tea, discontinue use. All herbs listed above are generally safe, though precautions should always be taken when using any type of medicine.*

Dual Purpose Tea

2 tsps dried German Chamomile flowers
1 cup boiling water

Steep the flowers in the boiling water, covered, for 15 minutes. Strain, then slowly sip the infusion to relieve nausea, stomach upset, and lessen menstrual cramps.

Do not drink more than 2 cups a day.

Echinacea & Roots Tea

A tasty way to help strengthen and support your natural resistance. A very popular tea.

1 pt Echinacea purpurea root
1 pt Pau d'Arco
1 pt Dandelion Root (raw and roasted)
1 pt Sarsaparilla bark
1 pt Cinnamon Bark
1 pt Ginger root
1 pt Burdock roots 1 pt Sassafras Bark a pinch of stevia

Place all herbs in a tea ball or bag and cover with boiling water. Steep for 10 minutes. Remove tea ball or bag, and add sugar, honey, sweetener, milk, cream or whatever, to taste.

End of Your Rope Tea

1 tbls. Chamomile
1 tbls. Peppermint

Put in a tea ball and steep in boiling hot water for five minutes.

Epilepsy Combination

1 tsp Valerian
1 tsp Skullcap
1 tsp Hops

Bring water to a boil and add herbs. Cover pot with lid and let steep for 5 minutes.

Evening Repose Tea

When the sun sets over the hill and the new moon dips her silver softness, savor the tranquility in our evening repose blend. It's a perfect toast to the rising moon. A robust flavor of flowers and mint.

1 pt Roses
1 pt Lavender flowers
1 pt Lemon Verbena leaves
1 pt Chamomile flowers
1 pt each Peppermint & Spearmint leaves
1 pt Blue Malva flowers pinch of stevia

Place all herbs in a tea ball or bag, and cover with boiling water. Steep for 10 minutes. Remove tea ball or bag, and add sugar, honey, sweetener, milk, cream or whatever, to taste.

❧ ✳ ☕ ✳ ❧

Feedee's Pain Killer Tea

The herbs you can choose from are as follows: **CHOOSE 5 TOTAL**

Lady's Mantle (herb)
Raspberry Leaf (herb)
Yarrow (herb)
Chaste Tree Berry
Fennel Seed (for the stomach)
Peppermint (for the stomach)
Valerian (for the stomach)

Use(1) part each (choose a total of five including one for the stomach).

Place all herbs in a tea ball or bag, and cover with boiling water. Steep for 5 to 10 minutes.
Remove tea ball or bag, and add sugar, honey, sweetener, milk, cream or whatever, to taste.

Fever Reducer Tea

2 tsp dried Catnip
1 tsp dry Vervain

Pour 2 cups boiling water over herbs. Steep 10 minutes & strain.

Fever Buster Tea

1 tbls. Catnip
1 tbls. White Oak Bark
1 tbls. Chamomile

Must be ingested as hot as the person can take it. Chamomile can be substituted for any other fragrant herb. It is added in only for taste.

Flashes Blend Tea

Brew up a pot and sip when needed.

1 pt Sage
1 pt Motherwort
1 pt Dandelion
1 pt Chickweed & violet leaves
1 pt each Elderflowers & Oatstraw

Place all herbs in a tea ball or bag, and cover with boiling water. Steep for 10 minutes. Remove tea ball or bag, and add sugar, honey, sweetener, milk, cream or whatever, to taste.

Flu-away

2 medium cloves of freshly crushed garlic
1 cup of very warm water
1 tsp of honey
1 tsp of Lemon juice

Stir and drink.

Fluid Retention Tea

1 oz Dandelion root
1 oz Dandelion leaves
2/3 oz Nettle Leaves
2/3 oz Spearmint leaves

Steep mixture in 1 cup of water for 10 minutes.

Happy Man Tea Blend

1 pt Siberian Ginseng
1 pt Dandelion Root
1 pt Nettle
1 pt each Marshmallow & Burdock roots
1 pt each Hawthorn & saw palmetto berries
1 pt Fennel Seeds 1 pt Wild Oats a pinch of stevia

Place all herbs in a tea ball or bag, and cover with boiling water. Steep for 10 minutes. Remove tea ball or bag, and add sugar, honey, sweetener, milk, cream or whatever, to taste. Climb into bed and enjoy!

Happy Tummy Tea

Put a smile on your face with this soothing and yummy tea.

1 pt Catnip
1 pt Spearmint & Lemongrass leaves
1 pt Calendula flowers
1 pt Skullcap
1 pt Rosemary & Sage leaves
1 pt Fennel Seeds

Place all herbs in a tea ball or bag, and cover with boiling water. Steep for 10 minutes. Remove tea ball or bag, and add sugar, honey, sweetener, milk, cream or whatever, to taste.

Headache Tea

1 pt Lavender
1 pt Chamomile
1 pt Rosemary
1 pt Mint

Put a pinch of each herb in a coffee filter and place in your coffee maker. Wait a half hour before drinking this mix, this should make you tired so you can sleep your headache away.

Healing Ginger tea

2 cups of water
4 tbls freshly grated Ginger root

Place in pan with a lid on, bring to a boil, turn off the heat and let sit for two hours. Reheat the tea, strain the herb from the tea and drink.

Health Is Wealth Tea

1 tbls. China black tea
2 tsp Fennel
1 tsp Mint
2 tsp Rose Hips
1 tsp Elderflower
2 tsp Hops
1 tsp Mullein

Place all herbs in a tea ball or bag, and cover with boiling water. Steep for 10 minutes. Remove tea ball or bag, and add sugar, honey, sweetener, milk, cream or whatever, to taste.

Heartburn Tea

1 tbls. Chamomile
1 tbls. Peppermint
2 pods Star Anise

Boil pods for 5 minutes and steep the chamomile and pepperMint in the Anise tea. Drink one cup every hour for two hours before bedtime.

Hops Sleep Blend

2 ounces Hops, dried
2 ounces of Chamomile, dried
1/2 ounce Eucalyptus leaves, dried
1 ounce Lemon Balm
1 ounce Orris Root powder
3 drops Lemon Balm essential oil

Bring water to a boil and add herbs. Cover pot with lid and let steep for 5 minutes.

Lady Tea

3 tbls. Sassafras Bark
2 tbls. Dandelion Root
1 tbls. Ginger root
½ tbls. Cinnamon
1 tbls. Licorice root
½ tbls. Orange Peel
1 tbls. Pau d'Arco
¼ tbls. Dong Quai root
1 tbls. Chaste Berry
1 tbls. Wild Yam

Place all herbs in a tea ball or bag, and cover with boiling water. Steep for 10 minutes. Remove tea ball or bag, and add sugar, honey, sweetener, milk, cream or whatever, to taste.

Forests Tea (formerly Lung Blend)

1 pt Echinacea purpurea
1 pt Elecampane
1 pt Ginger
1 pt each Pleurisy & Licorice roots
1 pt white Oak Bark
1 pt Cinnamon Bark
1 pt each Orange Peel and Fennel Seeds

Place all herbs in a tea ball or bag, and cover with boiling water. Steep for 10 minutes. Remove tea ball or bag, and add sugar, honey, sweetener, milk, cream or whatever, to taste.

❀ ✳ ☕ ✳ ❀

Indigestion Relief Tea

---

1 oz.   Chamomile
2/3 oz. Peppermint
1 oz.   Caraway Seeds
2/3 oz. Angelica

Use 1 tsp of the mixture per cup of hot water. Steep the mixture 10 min. and strain.

This tea soothes the gastrointestinal tract and stimulates digestive activity, making it useful for stomach aches or a too-full feeling

Insomnia Tea

1 ½ oz dried Vervain leaves
1 oz Chamomile
½ oz Spearmint

Mix all and add to 1 cup boiling water. Steep 8 minutes; strain.

Less Stress Tea

Relieves stress, relaxes low back and neck areas.

1 pt Chamomile
1 pt Mint
1 pt Calendula flowers

Place all herbs in a tea ball or bag, and cover with boiling water. Steep for 10 minutes. Remove tea ball or bag, and add sugar, honey, sweetener, milk, cream or whatever, to taste.

Mellow Mood Tea

This tea is made with the most palatable of the calming herbs.Blended together, they'll defuse stress and anxiety and promote sound sleep.

1 tsp Chamomile flowers
1 tsp Lavender spikes
1 tsp Kava leaves
1 tsp Lemon balm leaves
1 tsp Marjoram
1 spray Valerian flowers
1 quart water

In a large saucepan, steep the chamomile, lavender, Kava, lemon balm, marjoram, and valerian to taste in the freshly boiled water. Strain out the plant material. Drink the tea hot or cool as often as needed, refrigerating any left over for later use.

CAUTION: Chamomile is in the ragweed family, and can often causeallergic reactions.

❧ ✳ ☕ ✳ ❧

Memory Minder Tea

---

1 tsp Ginkgo Biloba
1 tsp Panax Ginseng
1 tsp Peppermint

Bring two cups of water to a boil. Add herbs and place a tight lid over the pot for five to ten minutes. Take one cup in the morning and one cup around mid-day.

Memory Zest Blend

A mentally refreshing beverage, to help give you feelings of clarity and precision.

1 pt Ginkgo
1 pt Gotu Kola and Peppermint leaves
1 pt Red Clover Tops
1 pt Rosemary leaves 1 pt Ginger root a pinch of stevia.

Place all herbs in a tea ball or bag, and cover with boiling water. Steep for 10 minutes. Remove tea ball or bag, and add sugar, honey, sweetener, milk, cream or whatever, to taste.

Migraine Tea

1 2/3 oz dried St John's Wort
1 oz Valerian
1 oz Linden flowers
1/4 oz Juniper berries

Use 1 tsp of mixture per 1 cup boiling water. Steep 10 minutes & strain.

Moon Ease Tea

For that time of the month.

2 pts Cramp Bark
1 pt Chaste Tree berries
1 pt each Spearmint & Skullcap leaves
1 pt Marshmallow root
1 pt Passionflower herb
1 pt Ginger root

Place all herbs in a tea ball or bag, and cover with boiling water. Steep for 10 minutes. Remove tea ball or bag, and add sugar, honey, sweetener, milk, cream or whatever, to taste.

My Nerves Are Shot Tea!

Uses:
Sleeplessness and Insomnia
Job-related stress
Panic attacks

2 pts Chamomile
1 pt Jasmine
1 pt Hops
1 pt Lavender
1 pt Yerba Santa
1 pt Gotu Kola
1 pt St. John's Wort

Place all herbs in a tea ball or bag, and cover with boiling water. Steep for 10 minutes. Remove tea ball or bag, and add sugar, honey, sweetener, milk, cream or whatever, to taste.

Natural Concentration Tea

Helps you to become more creative in designing a more natural environment in your home.

1 pt Calendula
1 pt Mint,
1 pt Sage (flowers only)
1 pt Yarrow Leaves

Place all herbs in a tea ball or bag, and cover with boiling water. Steep for 10 minutes. Remove tea ball or bag, and add sugar, honey, sweetener, milk, cream or whatever, to taste.

Nausea Tea

½ tsp dried Ginger root
½ tsp Clove blossoms
1 tsp Chamomile flowers

Pour 1 cup boiling water over herbs. Steep 10 minutes, strain & let cool.

Nervous Nancy Tea

1 ½ oz Peppermint leaves
1 ½ oz Lemon Balm leaves

Use 1 tsp of mixture per 1 cup boiling water. Steep 10 minutes &
strain.

Nervous Stomach Tea

2 tsp Angelica root
2 tsp Lemon Balm leaves
½ tsp Fennel seed

Bring Angelica root to a simmer in 4 cups of water. Turn off heat,add lemon balm & lemon; steep 10 minutes & strain.

Nervous Tension Tea

1 1/3 oz. St. John's Wort
1 oz. Lemon Balm Leaves
1 oz. Valerian

Use 1 tsp of the herb mixture per cup of boiling water. Steep for 10 min., strain, sweeten if necessary.

Drink a cup before going to bed each night for several weeks to calm nerves, lift depression, and help you fall asleep more easily.

"No-Sweat" Tea

4 cups boiling water
1 tsp. dried Hops
1 tsp. stinging Nettle
1 tsp. fresh cut Rose petals
1 tsp. dried Strawberry Leaves
1 tsp. fresh Walnut Leaves
3 tbsp of dried Sage leaves

Reduces perspiration within 2 hours of use with its effects lasting several days:

Combine all ingredients, cover and steep for an hour. Strain and sweeten with honey if desired.

Nursing Mother's Tea

1 tsp crushed Fennel Seeds
1 cup boiling water

Mix the seeds with the boiling water. Cover and steep for 10 minutes.Strain, and sip the infusion. Drinking a tea made with fennel helps to promote the secretion of breast milk in nursing mothers.

Pink Eye Tea recipe

1 pt Chamomile
1 pt Borag
1 pt Eyebright 1 pt Elderflowers.
5 drops Witch hazel extract
2 ½ cups boiling water

Fill a tea ball with equal parts:
chamomile(antiseptic), Borag (alleviated inflammation and redness),eyebright (excellent for conjunctivitis any other eye complaints), Elderflowers (beneficial for tired eyes).

Pour on 2 1/2 cups boiling hot water to allow it to steep until cooled. Add 5 drops witch hazel extract (coolant and antiseptic) and stir.

Wash around the outside of the eye gently with infusion. And put one drop of infusion in the eye as needed or desired. Also can be used by soaking a cloth in the infusion and putting over the eye until you eye feels better. This Is good for anything where your eyes are painful, inflamed and red.

***If you're using this for a child, leave out the witchhazel.

❀ ✳ ☕ ✳ ❀

Pleasant Dreams

---

1 cup Mugwort
1/2 cup Rose petals
1/2 cup Chamomile
1/3 cup Lavender flowers
1/3 cup Catnip
2 tbsp Mint

Place all herbs in a tea ball or bag, and cover with boiling water. Steep for 10 minutes. Remove tea ball or bag, and add sugar, honey, sweetener, milk, cream or whatever, to taste.

Quiet Child Tea

Good for anytime of the day or right before bedtime.

1 pt Raspberry leaves
1 pt Catnip
1 pt each Spearmint & Skullcap leaves
1 pt Calendula flowers a pinch of stevia

Place all herbs in a tea ball or bag, and cover with boiling water. Steep for 10 minutes. Remove tea ball or bag, and add sugar, honey, sweetener, milk, cream or whatever, to taste.

Quiet Time Tea

1 pt Oregano
2 pts Chamomile
1 pt Lemon balm
1 pt Lemon Thyme

Place all herbs in a tea ball or bag, and cover with boiling water. Steep for 10 minutes. Remove tea ball or bag, and add sugar, honey, sweetener, milk, cream or whatever, to taste.

Radiante YOU Tea

1 tsp honeybush leaves

Place honeybush leaves in a tea ball or bag, and cover with boiling water. Steep for 5 to 10 minutes. Remove tea ball or bag, and add sugar, honey, sweetener, milk, cream or whatever, to taste.

Honeybush tea is a pleasant way to keep the body well hydrated with fluids This herbal tea has many health benefits! Honeybush has nearly the same properties as Rooibos. It is caffeine free low in tannin, and very rich in antioxidants. It contains no additives, preservatives or colorants.

Honeybush has antispasmodic properties which means those with weak digestion can easily enjoy this tea. It has been a treatment for colic in babies. It also helps to relieve insomnia.

❧ ✳ ☕ ✳ ❧

Rapunzel Tea

---

1 tbls. Fenugreek (seeds, or leaves)
Honey to taste

Place all herbs in a tea ball or bag, and cover with boiling water. Steep
for 5 to 10 minutes.
Remove tea ball or bag, and add sugar, honey, sweetener, milk, cream
or whatever, to taste.

**Do not use if breastfeeding

Really Relaxing Tea

1 pt (1 tsp) Valerian root (dried)
1 pt (1 tsp) Chamomile flowers (dried)

In a Teapot pour in 2 mug fulls of hot water (not boiling) steep for 5 mins. Strain or remove tea bags. Add honey if desired. This is great at night before bed

❧ ✳ ☕ ✳ ❧

Rejuvenation Tea

Etheric cleanser of old, stale thoughts and patterns of behavior for new beginnings and awakening.

1 pt Rose Hips
1 pt Calendula flowers
1 pt Gallum (Cleavers) flowers
1 pt Borage flowers
1 pt Nettles leaves

Place all herbs in a tea ball or bag, and cover with boiling water. Steep for 10 minutes. Remove tea ball or bag, and add sugar, honey, sweetener, milk, cream or whatever, to taste.

Relaxation Tea

2 pts Chamomile
1 pt Lemon balm
1 pt Lemon peel
1 pt Thyme

Place all herbs in a tea ball or bag, and cover with boiling water. Steep for 10 minutes. Remove tea ball or bag, and add sugar, honey, sweetener, milk, cream or whatever, to taste.

Sleep Tea Recipe

2 tbls. Hops
1 tsp. Lavender
1 tsp. Rosemary
1 tsp. Thyme
1 tsp. Mugwort
1 tsp. Sage
1 Pinch of Valerian Root

Take a tsp of the mixture and pour into 1 cup of hot water. Let sit for 3 minutes then strain. Store the unused portion.

Soothing Tea

1 pt Mint
1 pt Hyssop
1 pt Oregano
1 pt Parsley
1 pt Lemon balm

Place all herbs in a tea ball or bag, and cover with boiling water. Steep for 10 minutes. Remove tea ball or bag, and add sugar, honey, sweetener, milk, cream or whatever, to taste.

Sore throat

1 tbls. Licorice root
1 tbls. Slippery Elm
1 tbls. Peppermint

Place all herbs in a tea ball or bag, and cover with boiling water. Steep for 10 minutes

Speakeasy (Bad Breath) Tea

1 tbls. Black, or Green tea leaves
1 tbls. Mint leaves
Honey to taste

Place all herbs in a tea ball or bag, and cover with boiling water. Steep for 5 to 10 minutes. Remove tea ball or bag, add honey to taste.

Antioxidants in the tea minimize bacteria that cause bad breath.

Spiced Relief

1 tsp. Anise Seeds, crushed or ground
2-3 Cinnamon sticks
1 inch of Ginger, sliced
1-2 tsp. dried loose Echinacea

Combine spices and Echinacea in a pot with three cups of water. Bring to a boil and then simmer for 15-20 minutes to make a decoction. Strain into a mug and add honey to taste.

This is a multifunction tea. Anise acts as an expectorant, Ginger soothes the cough, and cinnamon has antibacterial properties.

Stomach ache (Nausea)

Must be done in a pot on the stove.

1 pod of Star Anise per cup
1 pt Chamomile (bag or tea ball)

Combine ingredients in a pot with three cups of water. Bring to a boil and then simmer for 15-20 minutes to make a decoction. Strain into a mug and add honey to taste.

Stop that Cough Tea

1 tbls. Slippery Elm
1 tbls. Mullein
1 tbls. Catnip
1 tbls. Licorice root bark

Boil the bark first in two cups of water for 10 minutes. Place the rest of the herbs in a coffee filter and place the filter in a strainer. Strain the Licorice tea through the strainer into a mug and drink. Honey and lemon can be added.

❀ ✴ ☕ ✴ ❀

Stress-Reducing Rest up Tea

1/2 cup Sweet Hops
1/2 cup Mugwort
1/8 cup Sweet Marjoram

All the following recipes have the same measurements. Unless otherwise stated, they were brewed in a coffee maker or tea brewer.

Measurements: 1 tbls. of each type of herb
1 tbls. of honey to sweeten the tea

❁ ✳ ☕ ✳ ❁

Tranquility Tea

2 pts Red Clover Blossoms
2 pts Rose Hips
1 pt   German Chamomile flowers
1 pt   Peppermint leaves

Bring water to a boil and add herbs. Cover pot with lid and let steep
for 5 minutes.

❀ ✳ ☕ ✳ ❀

Tummy Tea

A wonderful tea blend to enjoy after a big meal or hectic day.

1 cup dried Peppermint
1 tbsp dried Rosemary
1 tsp dried Sage

Crush ingredients and mix well. Store in an airtight container. Steep 1 heaping tsp in a cup of boiling water for 1 minute. Sweeten with Honey.

Upset Stomach Tea

8 oz Peppermint leaves
8 oz Lemon Balm leaves
8 oz Fennel Seeds

Mix ingredients together. Store in an airtight container. Use 1 tsp of mixture per 1 cup boiling water. Steep 10 minutes; strain.

Urinary Infection Tea

1 tsp Uva Ursi
½ tsp each Corn Silk,
½ tsp Cramp Bark,
½ tsp Marshmallow root
½ tsp Rose Hips
1 quart water

Simmer herbs in water for a couple of minutes, then steep them for 20 minutes. Strain herbs.

Drink 2 to 4 cups daily. To make sure the infection is gone, continue taking the herbs for 2 days after the symptoms disappear.

Winter Tea

Boneset
Echinacea
Peppermint

Just use equal pts of each, or pre-made tea bags...3 bags, one of boneset, 1 of echinacea, and 1 of Peppermint.

Place all herbs in a tea ball or bag, and cover with boiling water. Steep for 10 minutes. Remove tea ball or bags, and add sugar, honey, sweetener, milk, cream or whatever, to taste.

Wise Woman Tea

A wonderful menopause tea. Gently calms, cools and balances.

1 pt Motherwort
1 pt Sage
1 pt Nettle Leaves
1 pt each Lemon balm & Mugwort leaves
1 pt Chaste Tree berries
1 pt Horsetail

Place all herbs in a tea ball or bag, and cover with boiling water. Steep for 10 minutes. Remove tea ball or bag, and add sugar, honey, sweetener, milk, cream or whatever, to taste.

❀ ✳ ☕ ✳ ❀

Sip to Wellness for a Better Life

Let these herbal tea remedies be just the beginning of your exploration into the incredible healing properties of natural herbs. Remember, food is not just sustenance; it's medicine. As you sip to wellness, savor each moment as a therapeutic experience, whether you're enjoying it alone in quiet reflection or sharing it with loved ones. Embrace the tranquility, and let the healing power of herbal tea nourish your body, mind, and soul. Here's to your continued journey towards wellness and the joy of discovering the endless wonders of natural remedies and healing foods.